MW01517825

Understanding Rapid Weight Loss Hypnosis

A Quickstart Guide To Lose Weight Naturally Fast Through Meditation Techniques, Hypnosis To Improve Mindful Eating

Self Help for Women Academy

The following Book is reproduced below with the goal of providing information that is as accurate and reliable as possible. Regardless, purchasing this Book can be seen as consent to the fact that both the publisher and the author of this book are in no way experts on the topics discussed within and that any recommendations or suggestions that are made herein are for entertainment purposes only. Professionals should be consulted as needed prior to undertaking any of the action endorsed herein.

This declaration is deemed fair and valid by both the American Bar Association and the Committee of Publishers Association and is legally binding throughout the United States.

Furthermore, the transmission, duplication, or reproduction of any of the following work including specific information will be considered an illegal act irrespective of if it is done electronically or in print. This extends to creating a secondary or tertiary copy of the work or a recorded copy and is only allowed with the express written consent from the Publisher. All additional right reserved.

The information in the following pages is broadly considered a truthful and accurate account of facts and as such, any inattention, use, or misuse of the information in question by the reader will render any resulting actions solely under their purview. There are no scenarios in which the publisher or the original author of this work can be in any fashion deemed liable for any hardship or damages that may befall them after undertaking information described herein.

Additionally, the information in the following pages is intended only for informational purposes and should thus be thought of as universal. As befitting its nature, it is presented without assurance regarding its prolonged validity or interim quality. Trademarks that are mentioned are done without written consent and can in no way be considered an endorsement from the trademark holder.

Table of Contents

Introduction

How to tolerate the urge to eat something that we should not eat? Meditation also helps us tolerate pain, visualize it, and let it go. Therefore, if you are trying to lose weight and you are faced with your favorite temptation, for example, a chocolate bar, take the following steps:

1. Look at the chocolate bar

2. Recognize it as a temptation, as something you would like to eat but would be an obstacle to your goals.

3. Visualize it as a wish and let it go away from you.

If you are going through a day full of anxieties, and you feel that at any minute, you will start eating without thinking, then practice meditative breathing, inhaling in four beats, holding in four beats, and exhaling in four beats.

This week we spoke with Patricio Lagos, yoga instructor, and director of the trends blog Ansia.cl. He gave us some recommendations to learn to meditate and to use meditation to control anxiety and appetite.

PL: All you need is the intention to want to do it, to give yourself the time and space for it. It is not a race or competition. It has to be done willingly, relax, and enjoy.

Yes, anyone can do it, and if you have trouble sitting on the floor for a while, don't worry, you can do it sitting in a chair. The main thing is to be comfortable and relaxed. Although you can meditate lying down, remember that the idea is not to sleep, but be present and attentive.

In your experience, what are the benefits of meditation, and how could it help you maintain a proper weight and avoid overeating?

PL: Meditation is a practice that helps you gain talent to guide the flow of your thoughts. If we talk about taking care of your weight and avoiding overeating, the state of relaxation that meditation produces will lower your anxiety level, leading to bad eating habits. After meditation, the mind is in a state of greater clarity, a state from which we are guided towards naturally beneficial behaviors for our body. When the mind is silenced, the wise voice of the body makes itself heard.

But: If we are trying to eat healthily and face a bar of chocolate or other temptation, how could meditation help us stay in line?

When meditation is done a constant practice, the clarity you get is also based on your decisions and habits of thought and behavior. Don't make chocolate or other temptation your enemy. You have to make peace with how things are because when you stop fighting, it is easier to move in the direction you want to go. Be patient with yourself. You are where you are supposed to be, and you are doing very well.

Give it a try, and you will see how meditation will help you control your weight!

Chapter 1.

Reasons We Feel Hungry

First of all, we have to understand the reasons why we are feeling hungry, since the actions to follow vary in each case; We can feel hungry for the following two reasons:

Insufficient Diet

When we do not have a balanced eating plan, which is very common in the famous "express diets" in which for some time you must consume only certain foods, our body stops receiving the necessary calories for its proper functioning.

An inadequate calorie intake motivates glucose levels to decrease. The brain detects this state of energy and will send the signal that we must eat to obtain more nutrients to be hungry.

It also happens when we include many simple carbohydrates in our diet, such as honey, sugar, desserts, cakes, flours.

Since these give our body a hit of glucose that is quickly depleted, this drop will make the brain detect the lack of glucose again and send the signal that we are hungry also.

Anxiety

When we are subjected to a lot of stress or our nerves are altered, we reach a state of anxiety. Anxiety causes our body to release a more significant amount of adrenaline. It interprets it as a sign of danger; By producing adrenaline, the basal metabolism is altered and causes us to burn a more significant number of calories and glucose.

By burning more glucose, we return to the point described above. The brain interprets this lack of energy and tries to compensate by making us eat more.

One of the leading causes of obesity today is anxiety; many people have problems controlling the emotions that occur in individual events in their life, such as when an important date is approaching, when they stop smoking, when they experience stressful situations at work, and this leads them to binge-eat.

What to Do to Control Hunger?

First, we must clarify an important point. Suppose you are following a diet to lose weight. In that case, it is common for you to feel some hunger since to reduce your weight, you need to consume fewer calories than your body uses. However, nutritionists consider this factor and will recommend some snacks that you can introduce to satisfy your cravings without breaking your plan.

It is why it is not advisable to follow diets without a prior professional evaluation. You could be causing a state of anxiety in your body that interferes with your goals and mainly with your health.

If you are eating correctly but still feeling hungry shortly after eating, here are some recommendations.

Include Foods That Promote Satiety

The best strategy is to include in our meals some foods that promote the feeling of satiety but that at the same time do not have a caloric intake as high as to interfere with our objectives; some options are the following:

The nuts are a rich source of fiber, which will make us feel full longer because it is processed very slowly in the body.

They have some fats, but these are mainly good fatty acids that help control blood cholesterol levels. About 50 grams of nuts in snacks will help to control hunger effectively.

Another food that has been popularly used to control hunger is an apple; it contains pectin and fiber that, in combination, help create satiety without forgetting that the apple is a rich source of vitamins.

The lemon has the quality thanks to its acidity keeps controlled cravings for sweet foods, which are the ones we make you fat.

Green leafy vegetables are high in water and fiber. The latter has already been mentioned as essential to generating satiety. Add little hot spices or chili to your food.

The spiciness helps stimulate the metabolism, giving us the feeling of being satisfied for longer after eating. The eggs are high in protein, which will also make us feel full longer.

The mint tea is also a vital ally to control hunger, as this herb interferes directly in the digestive processes. A cup of tea between meals or after meals can keep your anxiety to eat in check.

Eat some fat and carbohydrates; while this may sound against your goal of losing weight, the truth is that the body needs those doses of energy to keep its glucose production in check.

Go for complex carbohydrates like whole grains. In the case of fats, they help the body release a leptin hormone that keeps hunger in check; we do not recommend that you eat junk food, but some low-fat foods throughout the day will be beneficial for managing anxiety.

Another recommendation is to drink enough water; on many occasions, we confuse our brain's signals and think that we are hungry when, in fact, we are thirsty.

When you think you are hungry, have a glass of water. If you still feel hungry after a few minutes, it is convenient to consume some food like the ones we mentioned above.

Water should be part of your diet since it will help you control hunger and anxiety and eliminate toxins. Accumulated fat in your body, do not forget that the daily recommendation is eight glasses.

Chapter 2.

Meal Replacement Diets: Risks and Benefits

What to do to lose them? Can we choose to use meal replacements?

According to specialists in endocrinology and nutrition, it is not usually the most appropriate, and the doctor must always control its intake to avoid nutritional problems.

"It's improper or uncontrolled consumption can lead to nutritional imbalances, such as loss of muscle mass; metabolic, such as hypoglycemia, alteration of the acid-base balance or deficiency of vitamins and minerals; and lack of hydro-electrolytes, such as iron deficiency or water depletion."

It adds that it can also decompensate chronic diseases, such as kidney, liver, and heart failure. "For this reason, it is important that its use is regulated and medically supervised." An opinion shared by Andrea Calderón, dietician nutritionist and scientific secretary of the Spanish Society of Dietetics and Food Sciences (Seca): "Most of them are unhealthy products, of low nutritional interest and very expensive," he says.

Ingredients with Low Contribution

According to Calderón, simple sugars prevail among its ingredients, especially fructose, proteins of low nutritional quality "and sometimes in deficient quantity" and refined flours or starch from them. "Although these products are enriched with enough vitamins and minerals to cover daily needs, something that is not always met, they do not become better options because their base ingredients are not good," he warns.

For all these reasons, the doctor's indications must always be followed, related to the nutritional regimen that will accompany the substitutes and the duration.

And he adds: "Special attention must be paid to the total protein intake, to avoid protein deficiency in all cases, although it is especially harmful if the patient is preparing for surgery since protein malnutrition increases the risk of postoperative complications."

Where Is Your Job Most Beneficial?

In some specific situations, the use of meal replacement products may be helpful. For example, they are an exciting option when rapid weight loss is required before bariatric surgery, mainly treating morbid obesity.

"Its use has shown clinical benefits, such as reduction of the risk of surgical complications and recovery time after the intervention; increased odds of choosing a laparoscopic technique versus open surgery; shorter intervention time; and greater ease for the surgical approach, fundamentally derived from the reduction of the size of the liver," enumerates the spokesperson of the SEEN.

It ensures that cases have been described. The use of very-low-calorie diets based on meal replacement products has been associated with more significant weight loss after surgery. "And also, with an increase in patient adherence to nutritional and lifestyle changes after the intervention.

However, all this must be confirmed with other studies that include a greater number of patients."

Who Is It More Harmful to?

The use of these products is not recommended in children, adolescents, pregnant and lactating women. "They are not recommended either in people over 65 years of age and in people with certain diseases such as advanced kidney failure, severe liver failure, severe heart failure, severe depression, and psychiatric illnesses," says García.

For the rest, as has already been explained, its use is not suitable and can have a series of long-term adverse effects. According to the Seca specialist, its uncontrolled use can put an overload on the liver. "Without forgetting that if we continually opt for these products in cycles, we will drive our metabolism crazy and have a greater risk of rebound effect and of gaining body fat," he warns.

The best way to lose weight safely, according to Calderón, is through healthy lifestyle habits. "You have to plan a diet based on foods adapted to each person's circumstances, which can be balanced in a thousand ways according to the taste, possibilities, and preferences of each one, and without having to resort to substitutes," he explains.

And he adds: "Always accompanied by sufficient physical activity and an active life, two great forgotten reasons why many people consider that they cannot lose weight, but that they would be the solution in most cases."

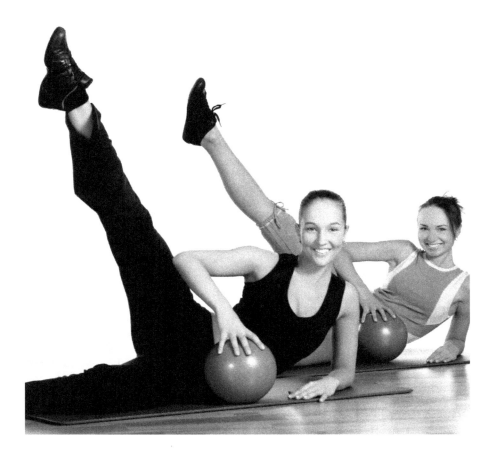

Chapter 3.

Chrono Nutrition and Chronobiology

Eat Everything, but at the Right Time

More than a diet, it is a diet that recommends following the body's metabolic rhythms, believing that food produces different effects depending on the moment it is eaten. Ideal for losing weight, but also for regaining physical and mental well-being. Think about it, an email that arrives at 3 in the morning produces a different effect than when it comes at 3 in the afternoon, annoyance or rejection. In the best of cases, it is ignored.

It is also what happens to our body when it "receives" certain foods at "wrong" times of the day, explains Prof. Fabio Rinaldi, Professor of Dermatology at the University of Brescia, Florence, Paris, and President of the International Hair Research Foundation.

But wrong for whom?"For the metabolic rate of that particular moment, afternoon, night, or morning." A practical example to explain that, as some dieticians also explain, yes, it is necessary to eat everything but choosing the right moments throughout the day.

It is the concept based on "Chrono nutrition," or that food science was born in 1986 from the studies of Dr. Delabos and that, explains Prof.

Rinaldi, "it is not a dietary regime in a restrictive sense, but a food control that takes into account not only what you eat but when you eat it, based on the changes in the body's metabolism at various times of the day, regulated by the circadian rhythm which oversees many of the vital functions, starting with the sleep-wake cycle."

To make our body function at its best, it is necessary to follow its rhythms, such as metabolic and hormonal changes and Chrono nutrition, matching food and nutritional needs to these rhythms during the 24 hours, from midnight to midnight. We then asked Dr. Rinaldi to explain how metabolism works and how a day should be addressed and "divided" from a food perspective.

How Does the Metabolic Rate Work?

"The most important part of the day is in the morning between 7 and 8 and at night, which is not a useless moment of the day but fundamental for the metabolism."

How should a typical food scheme be composed?

"Assuming that the same food produces different effects depending on the time it is eaten, in the morning between 7 and 8 the metabolic activity is at its maximum and, at this time, everything we eat is highly digested and metabolized. It is why you should never skip breakfast, which must be consumed by 8 am because hormones such as insulin, which controls the level of sugars, and cortisol, which affects blood pressure, reach their peak at this time.

The ideal would be to consume the typical breakfast with biscuits, milk, and coffee, which includes carbohydrates, fats, and sugars, excellent for giving energy because at this moment, the batteries need to be recharged, and everything is consumed faster."

At lunch?

"Towards the middle of the day, between 12 and 13, thyroid hormones rise, accelerating metabolism and preventing fat from accumulating. In this period, i.e., during lunch, we need carbohydrates, such as pasta, rice, bread, potatoes to combine with vegetables or legumes, because the thyroid needs the energy to function."

Fats and sugars for breakfast, carbohydrates for lunch, and in the evening?

"Beyond personal habits (you don't eat or eat little), dinner should be eaten between 7 pm and 8 pm and always by 10 pm, when there is an increase in growth hormone and somatostatin that stimulate formation muscle tissue and tissue regeneration in general.

Therefore, favoring the increase in lean mass. It is then the right time to eat proteins, such as meat, fish, or legumes, with a high protein value and limit carbohydrates because insulin has slowed down. Therefore, sugars are assimilated more easily."

It is also the time when the body prepares for the night and before bed; recommends Dr. Rinaldi, "it is good to take herbal teas but not fruit, for example, rich in sugars that are badly assimilated because the insulin level is low."

One exception: the banana, which is rich in tryptophan, stimulates the synthesis of melatonin, thus promoting sleep. "A banana very rich in tryptophan has a very different action whether it is eaten at nine in the morning or nine in the evening," says Dr. Rinaldi.

But what if you can't follow the eating pattern?

"Variations can be introduced, but small. You can move lunch or dinner a little, but there must always be a period of a few hours between meals. Also, we can allow ourselves some tears in the regime, which must be balanced either in the next meal or the day after."

Are there any foods to avoid?

«In principle, no, everything must be assumed. Perhaps it would be better to limit those with inflammatory action, rich in histamine such as milk and derivatives or vegetables, such as aubergines, tomatoes, peas, and then the foods with preservatives, additives, glutamates. In principle, rather than eliminating food, it is necessary to select the foods.»

Can cosmetic products containing the same active ingredients as foods help or favor their action?

"More than anything else, they can promote skin hydration, but usually the opposite happens: we treat skin and hair problems with the right nutrition." And here, Chrono nutrition becomes Chrono dermatology or Chrono cosmetics, in the words of a dermatologist!

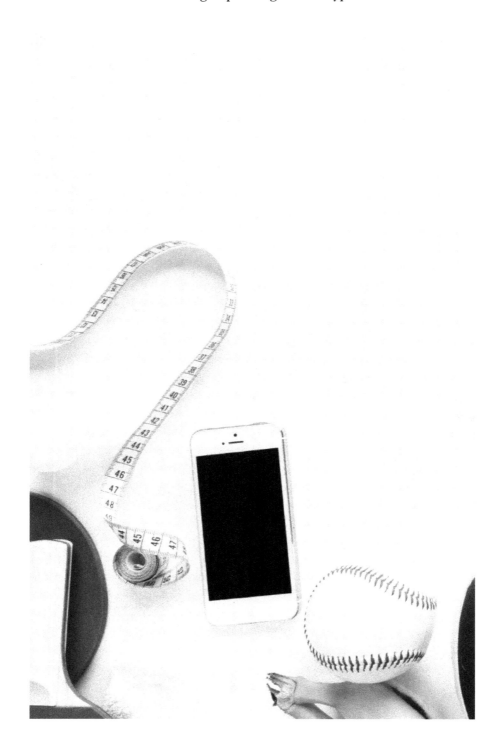

Chapter 4.

Diet, Here Is the Right Time to Eat

Recent research that appeared in the latest issue of Cell Metabolism brings exciting advice for those who want to lose weight, beyond the specific diet that you choose to undertake (remember, always and only after talking to your doctor!

A team of scholars led by researcher Joseph Takahashi discovered that it is essential to understand and evaluate what and how much we eat and the "when," that is, the moment in which our body consumes calories. In this sense, Takahashi stated that a diet is only beneficial if the calories are consumed during the day when we are awake and active.

The study points out that circadian rhythms regulate the sleep-wake cycle and affect how we store or consume calories, burn sugars, develop fat, and so on.

All these parameters fluctuate to a considerable extent during the day. Therefore, being able to eat in harmony with these cycles allows food to be metabolized with fewer problems.

More specifically, the research suggests proceeding with a relatively abundant breakfast and then gradually reducing individual meals' contributions to arrive at a light dinner, easily assimilated by the body.

Lunch must instead be more substantial than dinner to ensure our body remains active.

By following this simple rule, it is, therefore, possible to maximize our well-being: eating in the furthest possible moments from when you go to sleep should be a good source of inspiration to be active and burn calories more efficiently.

Having said that, if you want to undertake a diet, we can only advise you to talk carefully with your doctor and identify with him the right path to follow

When Is the Right Time To Eat?

When it comes to mealtimes, cultural, family, and personal habits are the most varied: to put some order between traditions, stereotypes, and "hearsay" today.

Let's see what the right time to eat according to Chinese medicine is.

The principle on which we will talk about is based on the fact that the circulation of qi ("energy") and healthy qi, called yangqin, follows a precise order and rhythm.

In fact, according to Chinese medicine, qi flows following a nictemeral cycle (24 hours) within the 12 main meridians: this flow, therefore, affects the system of organs and viscera c (which is the basis of the functioning of our organism) thanks to their direct connection with the meridians.

Obviously, qi ("energy") must be present everywhere at all times to ensure nourishment, protection, processing, communication, heating to all parts of the body, and then allow our lives. Still, this ongoing stream has minimums and maximums for each organ or bowel, depending on the time of day.

To better understand this concept, just think of the rivers, seas, and oceans of the Earth: even if they have different names, they are part of a single circuit, and therefore, they are all connected.

Although water is always present at all times in all points of the course, the seas and oceans have high and low tide movements, which occur at specific times. These movements are so important that even the great rivers are affected.

In the same way, the main meridians (those connected directly to the organs and viscera) form a circuit always covered by qi ("energy"), which, however, is more cyclically present in a specific meridian than the others (maximum energy).

Twelve hours later, qi is less present in the same meridian (energy minimum). This tidal wave runs through the entire meridian circuit in 24 hours: given that, there are 12 meridians. It can be deduced that the maximum energy (and the minimum energy 12 hours later) will last two hours for each meridian.

The Right Time to Eat, to Sleep, to Work

Since this energetic tidal wave affects all meridians and, therefore, all organs and viscera, we can understand when each of them is at its maximum activity and when it is at its minimum to regulate our lifestyle more healthily suitably.

So, let's see how the flow of qi moves in the 24 hours, to understand not only what is the right time to eat, but also the most suitable time to rest, to do physical activity, to relate to others, etc.

From 5 to 7: the right time for meditation and bath. From 5 to 7, the large intestine is at its maximum energy: the most immediate reflection is that this is undoubtedly the best time to go to the bathroom. The lung (which takes care of bringing the air inside and outside the body and, therefore, directing qi's movement, "energy" in general) has already started to stimulate our activation from 3 in the morning. In the time slot linked to the large intestine, we are therefore ready to activate bowel movements.

However, for this to happen, it is necessary to have some time and relaxation: it is better to get up 5 minutes earlier to remain quiet in the bathroom rather than do everything in a hurry and compromise the emptying of the intestine.

According to Chinese medicine, the metal element (which includes lung and large intestine) is also linked to introspection. This time slot is the most suitable for meditating or engaging in physical practices based on breathing (lung) such as yoga and qigong. If you suffer from constipation, it may help to practice one of these activities as soon as you wake up to get your qi moving with breathing and then go to the bathroom.

In addition to this, I suggest you read my article dedicated to the topic: Constipation in pregnancy (and not only): a practical remedy. The lung is at its minimum energy between 15 and 17: indeed, this is the least suitable time slot for physical activity. From 7 to 9: the right time to eat a critical meal.

The stomach is at its maximum energy between 7 and 9 in the morning: this means that its qi ("energy") is at its maximum, and this bowel can receive, grind and pass down even the most foods. "Difficult." From 9 to 11, it's up to the spleen: according to Chinese medicine, the energy function of this organ is complementary to that of the stomach because it is responsible for selecting and absorbing the useful components (in Chinese medicine, they say "pure," therefore usable) of food and the drinks that the stomach has amalgamated and reduced to pulp.

Therefore, the time slot from 7 to 9 is the right time to eat to capture the stomach's energy peak and, subsequently, the spleen.

We deduce that (as we often hear) breakfast should be the most critical meal because it is the moment when the stomach and spleen can maximize digestion and metabolization of food. In a nutshell, we can draw more useful substances from food and drink, consuming less qi to do so and leaving only the waste to go to the intestines.

Suppose this topic sends you into crisis, and you want to understand how to seize the right time to eat at this time slot. In that case, I suggest you read my article "What to eat for breakfast? 5 tips to stay healthy all day," with lots of practical information.

On the contrary, between 7 pm and 11 pm, the stomach and spleen are at their minimum energetic: our dinner, therefore, takes place in an incredibly tricky time slot for these organs, which is not precisely the right time to eat to maintain a good balance of the system digestive (and not only!) we should have a light meal and not too late.

From 1 PM to 3 PM: The Afternoon Nap

In the time slot between lunch, the small intestine is at its energetic maximum. At this moment, our energies should be dedicated to the absorption and assimilation phase of the nutrients and liquids present in the chyme that has passed from the stomach into the small intestine.

Chinese medicine says that this bowel deals with "separation." If the spleen does the bulk of assimilating nutrients, the small intestine is significant because it must filter in an even more refined way from the stomach.

During these two hours, it would therefore be an excellent idea to let the small intestine work without consuming too much qi ("energy") for other activities: an afternoon nap or rest would be ideal. In this context, physical activity is not recommended, also because, at this moment, the liver is at its minimum energy and cannot perform at its best its action of distributing blood to the muscles

From 1 to 3: Deep Sleep

In this time slot, the energetic tidal wave arrives in the liver meridian. According to Chinese medicine, this organ is responsible for promoting and making qi fluid circulation, distributing blood where needed (depending on its activity). It draws the blood to itself (in Chinese medicine, it is said "Blood warehouse") to regenerate it.

Between 1 am and 3 am, sleep must be in its most in-depth phase: in this way, the body completely at rest will not need to receive large quantities of blood, which can be recalled by the liver. The sense organ linked to the liver is the eyes; thus, watching TV or reading/studying during this time slot is not recommended.

According to Chinese medicine, the liver is also linked to dreams, both nocturnal and "with open eyes": resting deeply at this time allows us to keep our planning and design skills active.

Indicative Time Slots, Not the Bible!

An important note on the circulation of qi in the meridian circuit: the rhythm described can be taken as defined and fixed if our schedules are regular and if we follow the rhythm of nature to carry out our activities.

In other words, the farmer who gets up with the sun, follows the rhythms "of the past," and goes to bed early can take these time slots literally.

Still, those with a completely different rhythm should take them as an indication.

We can therefore rely on the table to draw these conclusions:

- It is essential to respect morning bowel regularity and to take time to breathe as soon as you wake up.

- Breakfast must be well fed and balanced, while dinner must be light and straightforward.

- The moment after lunch should not be overloaded with physical and mental activity.

- It's best to go to bed as soon as possible.

We also consider that we have daylight saving time: 9 pm in reality in Italy in the summer. The sun's movement is 8 pm. Dine a little later than in winter (to take advantage of the hours of light) is, therefore, less dramatic than it might seem.

"Breakfast like a king, lunch like a prince, dinner like a poor man."

Popular Saying:

The right time to eat, but also the right way.

Breakfast

From this overview, we understood that the most critical moment of the day for our nutrition is the morning: it is the right time to eat par excellence. The breakfast, which we often neglect, should instead be a complete and decadent meal to devote the proper time sitting at the table.

However, the time is essential for a good breakfast and what you eat: the typical Italian breakfast, based on dairy products, sweets, and white flour products, is certainly not the most suitable. It is for two main reasons:

According to the correspondences of the five elements, the sweet taste is connected to the stomach-spleen system, which deals with digestion. Small quantities of natural sweet taste (cereals, fruit, vegetables such as pumpkin or potato) supports and fortifies it, while an excessive amount of sweet taste (especially if "extreme" like that of sugar or honey) makes it difficult—that is to say, "too much is good."

Milk and dairy products, white flours and derivatives, sugar and sweets are humectant foods: this means that they are incredibly heavy and "clogging" (such as humidity, which impregnates the tissues making them heavy and causes walls and ceilings to swell), so the stomach and spleen they cannot fully assimilate them. The amount of qi required to process them is more generous than average, and this weakens the digestive system and hinders the assimilation of useful ("pure") substances.

However, to start on the right foot, it would be better to favor preparations based on grains such as muesli or oat flakes, wholemeal bread, fruit, dried fruit, and oilseeds (walnuts, hazelnuts, almonds, pumpkin seeds, seeds of sunflower), sources of proteins (from ham to eggs to hummus, according to your tastes), vegetable kinds of milk in small quantities.

Since the stomach and spleen are at their maximum energy at this moment, even small quantities of wet food are better tolerated: depending on your taste, you can add a little yogurt, cheese, a slice of cake, or a piece of focaccia.

The essential thing is to vary your breakfast within the week (each flavor has a precise relationship with our balance.

Therefore, the best key is variety) and according to the seasons (how we change clothes and habits to conform to environmental changes).

Lunch

Even if the right time to eat everything that needs to give us energy during the day is in the morning, it is still a substantial meal. Lunch must support us during the afternoon work: skipping it would be a mistake because it would lead us to arrive at dinner very hungry.

Grain cereals (rice, spelled, barley, quinoa) accompanied by vegetables or proteins (meat, fish, legumes) are ideal because they support the formation of qi ("energy") and therefore are well spendable and long-lasting.

If it's hot and you want to eat a fresh salad, prepare it by mixing vegetables, cereals, legumes (peas or lentils, mostly if peeled, they are more digestible than beans), seeds, and a source of protein if you haven't already used legumes (egg, tuna, a small amount of cheese such as feta or parmesan).

You will not be weighed down, and you will have everything necessary to produce the qi that will support you in the second part of the day.

Dinner

For us, it is a meal with significant social and emotional value: a frugal dinner in itself makes us sad. However, we must not think to have a light dinner.

You have to give up taste: the first step is to eliminate from feed (or strongly reduce) wet foods (baked goods, flour derivatives such as pasta, milk and dairy products, large quantities of fruit, desserts) and focus on recipes prepared with the other foods.

Since it is not the right time to eat, not compromising the rest of the night (and not to require an excessive delivery of qi and blood to the stomach), it is also better to avoid heavy cooking such as frying. The momentary exception is not a problem, but the important thing is the rule!

So, what to eat for dinner? The meal has to be varied according to the season. Still, the ideal elements are vegetables (better if cooked, especially in winter) and purees, creams or soups, small quantities of grains, legumes, fish, occasionally eggs.

Tasty and straightforward examples are an anchovy pie with aromatic herbs, capers, and grated Parmesan cheese (write me if you want the recipe) accompanied by steamed vegetables, sautéed, stewed, or raw (in summer) or a chickpea soup with the addition of clams and toasted wholemeal bread.

As you may have noticed, for the evening meal, many foods are strongly discouraged that DIY diets are used to replace dinner: yogurt, salad, fruit, mozzarella do not lighten us, but they weigh us down! Much better to eliminate wet foods from feed and as much as possible from the rest of the day: this will avoid further accumulations and dispose of those present.

The Right Time to Eat: Change Habits Gradually

If your habits are entirely different, it may be easier for you to gradually change them to use the right time to eat (i.e., in the morning) to recharge your batteries. An excellent way to start is to have an afternoon snack and significantly reduce the amount of what you eat for dinner, choosing to go to bed a little earlier than usual. In this way, you will wake up with a clear stomach and a better appetite, and it will be easier to think about having a big breakfast.

Even a different arrangement with lunch may not be comfortable, especially if you are out. The offer of bars and restaurants is not significantly varied.

A useful suggestion is to cook something for dinner that you can assemble differently for lunch: if you make a legume and cereal soup, you can cook spelled separately, adding it to the soup when cooked and using part of it for lunch. The next day, just add a source of protein, a handful of seeds, some cooked vegetables, or diced tomatoes if it's summer, and your lunch will be ready to go with minimal effort.

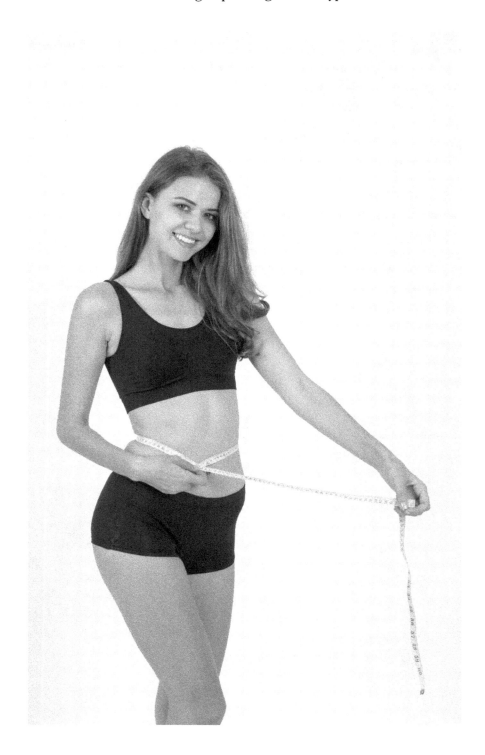

Chapter 5.

What Are the Foods to Avoid and Never Eat?

Balance and variety are two concepts that I will repeat until you have them well marked in your mind. Proportions of the single dish, vegetables in abundance, whole grains, proteins and healthy fats, no excesses: these are the general indications that I offer every time we talk about healthy nutrition. Scientific societies and guidelines suggest the same food.

However, every day we are bombarded with information of all kinds and origins. Distinguishing valid ones from those with the same scientific basis as fried air can also become very complicated for a non-expert.

Even with the knowledge necessary to eat at their best, there is still the danger of being overwhelmed by crafty food marketing campaigns: on the other hand, the ultimate purpose of companies is to sell their product, even if it is right to mention their increasing attention to the real needs of the population in the formulation of food.

Therefore, it becomes all too easy to get confused about which foods we can define as healthy and which are not.

How important are the methods of farming and cultivation, transport, storage, and cooking?

We have learned that more food is consumed as it is, the better it will be for our health. Buying fish, fruit, and vegetables at the market, meat from the trusted butcher, eggs, cheese and milk from the farmer, and wholemeal flours from a mill should be everyone's favorite choice in an ideal world.

Joining a local product-buying group can be a viable solution (and certainly more feasible than the previous one). However, the reality is that most of the city population finds themselves on Saturday morning in the chaos of parking lots, special offers, and unmissable promotions of the various shopping centers to do the "big shopping."

Therefore, it becomes necessary to learn to extricate yourself among the supermarket shelves, to try to put the equivalent of a healthy diet in our shopping carts.

Of course, an inevitable fact must be taken into account: a tomato sold in neat plastic trays will never have the same characteristics (nutritional, texture, taste, and smell) as one just picked from the plant, and so for most products.

Technology allows us to have foods that retain the same characteristics as fresh ones, or almost. Globalization makes South American oranges available to us at lower costs than Sicilian ones.

But at what price?

Unfortunately, the price is given by nutritional content that is, in many cases, decreased compared to local or non-preserved products: let's see how much this can affect our diet.

The substances that interest us in food and which can undergo variations based on various factors are macronutrients (proteins, carbohydrates, and fats), micronutrients (vitamins and mineral salts), fibers, and phytochemicals (flavonoids, carotenoids).

The macronutrients may vary mainly because of cultivation and breeding methods. Type of land, cultivation, and harvesting times in agriculture determine some differences: an example is a difference in the carbohydrate content of a fruit concerning its ripeness (an apple picked at the right time will be sweeter than an unripe one due to its higher sugar content).

The types of farming and the feed used can determine differences in the quality of fats and the final organoleptic characteristics of the foods, such as fish, meat, eggs, and milk.

The different types of storage do not significantly affect the original macronutrient contents. However, the intake of fats or sugars of products preserved in oil or water (in cans), or the percentage of water in dried foods, will vary.

Transport has a little effect while cooking can make nutrients more digestible, as in egg proteins (soft-boiled or scrambled egg) or potato carbohydrates.

The fibers vary mainly due to the preparation methods: for example, a fruit and vegetable juice breaks the fibers, reducing the work for us and our digestive system (and the consequent benefit from their intake). The extracts altogether remove the thread from the final product.

The contents of vitamins, mineral salts and phytochemicals change a lot starting from cultivation methods (traditional or organic), harvest times, farming methods and animal feed, product treatment (such as pasteurization), conservation (deep freezing, modified atmosphere), and the cooking method.

In particular, many vitamins (especially vitamin C) decrease with time due to exposure to heat and air. At the same time, the mineral salts are dispersed when boiled in water.

In some cases, cooking proves positive in activating some protective components, such as lycopene in tomatoes' peel. Still, it destroys vitamin C or allows the elimination of some antinutrients, such as phytates of legumes and cereals.

What to do then?

The best thing is to choose less processed foods from short supply chains or zero km, alternate the types of preparation and consumption of cooked and raw foods, and choose less aggressive cooking methods, such as stewing and steaming.

Is it true that vegan and raw food diets allow you to eat healthier foods?

Suppose we had to summarize the indications on a diet as much as possible. In that case, the two main ones could be consuming many vegetables and foods that have undergone as few technological processes as possible. Son the spot, apparently perfect answers are veganism and raw food. Without going into the merits of the ethical convictions underlying these legitimate choices, it must be said that being vegan or raw food does not ensure healthiness and health.

There are many highly processed products allowed in vegan diets, such as protein substitutes. But even fries are vegan, yet they are not healthy. In this case, attention must be placed on searching for quality, reading the labels, and consuming all the nutrients necessary for a healthy diet. In the case of raw food, the issue is complicated because the danger is to eliminate entire categories of food, that is all those cooked over 40 degrees: to eliminate pasteurized milk, many kinds of cheese, many portions of meat, and vegetables that cannot be eaten raw, cereals and legumes. So be careful in choosing particular dietary regimes that are best for us.

Chapter 6.

Sleep and Health: Useful Tips for Better Sleep

Sleep is a decisive factor for our health: resting deeply for at least 6-7 hours a night is essential to maintain good health and psychophysical efficiency.

What Damages on Our Organism?

Scientific research has verified how great the impact that lacks or lack of sleep has on our bodies. Sleeping less than six hours exposes us to the risk of gaining weight and having accidents of all kinds, increases anxiety and depression, lowers our immune defenses, increases the risk of developing severe chronic diseases, such as diabetes, arthritis, breast cancer, lung diseases, gastroesophageal reflux disease, thyroid dysfunction, Parkinson's disease and Alzheimer's.

Lack of sleep is also associated with diseases affecting the heart and brain tissue and memory, and fertility.

Furthermore, an inability to recover appropriately prevents our cells from regenerating and renewing themselves, causing us to age prematurely.

Helpful Tips for a Restorative Sleep

The best hours for night rest are those ranging from 22.00 to 6.00 / 7.00 in the morning in compliance with the natural sleep-wake cycle dictated by sunlight for millennia.

The best quality of sleep, another fundamental element for our health, depends a lot on our habits.

It would be preferable to avoid:

- Decadent dinners after 20-20.30

- Take meat in the evening

- Stay connected to the internet and use a pc or smartphone after 9 pm

- Practice physical activity for strength in the late evening

- On the contrary, it is advisable:

  - Light dinners based on vegetables and fish

  - Deep breathing when walking in the fresh air

  - Listening to emotional music

The last decisive element to determine a good quality of rest is, as always, physical activity, which should be mainly aerobic and practiced daily. People who practice regular physical activity, in fact, rest better, enjoy a night of deep and restorative sleep, and fall asleep easier.

Habits Against Fatigue: Ideal Routine

It has happened to everyone to wake up in the morning feeling very tired, almost as if the previous night hadn't passed. The hours of rest have died in vain, and in the end, we don't feel rested at all. Some healthy anti-fatigue habits can help us tackle this problem.

Some factors make the time we devote to rest ineffective. The secret to sleeping well and not wake up tired has its roots in concentration.

It may seem like a paradox, but we need to focus on what we are doing: sleep. It and other anti-fatigue habits will make us more active and productive.

Dinner is another crucial factor. The popular belief that consuming fatty foods in the evening promotes nightmares has something to do with it. Because of an embolism risk following slow digestion, the body sends alarms to avoid falling into such a deep sleep and risk dying.

Achieving a state of complete relaxation is possible. For this, we must use some natural products, relaxation techniques and establish a healthy routine. It will help our brain recognize that it's time to go to bed.

Today we will talk about some tricks or habits against fatigue to include in your routine. They will help you feel more energetic.

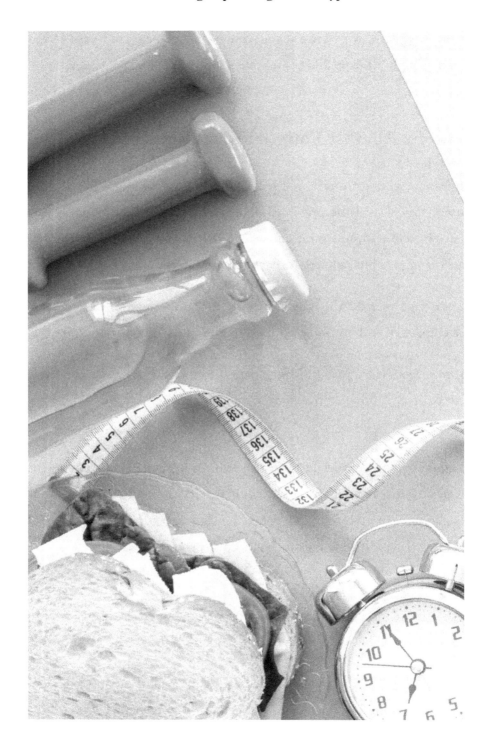

Chapter 7.

Sleeping Is Good for Your Health

March 15 is World Sleep Day 2019: this year, it is characterized by the slogan 'Healthy sleep, healthy aging,' underlining the fundamental influence of the quality of rest on our general health. Perdormire's commitment and the ten rules to rest well and for proper sleep hygiene.

Sleeping well is just as important as breathing. That's why the Twelfth World Day of sleep this year is characterized by the slogan 'Healthy sleep, healthy aging' (a sound sleep for healthy living), to emphasize the fundamental influence of the quality of rest on our overall health. Sleep disorders, from bad habits to pathologies, affect our well-being, and are also a public health problem.

To sleep, among the bedding sector's protagonists, consciously assumes in its corporate mission the responsibility, intrinsic in its activity: to produce mattresses, one of the main tools that determine the good sleep quality.

Therefore, it participates in the promotion of World Sleep Day. After all, the Materassificio Montalese—the PerDormire brand owner—is strongly committed to innovation and research and development. The target? Improving the quality of mattresses by implementing new technologies, such as AIIR Technology or the brand new Octaspring Project, is about to revolutionize the mattress market: two innovations added to the more than 20 proprietary patents of the company.

Moreover, PerDormire associates technology with innovative materials, such as BIO ones, based on soy and with essential vegetable seed oils, or fabrics that incorporate microcapsules with aloe essence, release their beneficial principles upon contact with the body. Materials and technologies that, in synergy with other characteristics, satisfy each person's comfort request. Yes, because concerning the mattress, everyone has their own unique ergonomic needs related to the physical constitution, thermal sensitivity, allergic predispositions, and other factors. To ensure this consumer need, PerDormire uses a technology that maps the comfort of the products; the Ergo Check test—with 648 sensors—analyzes the pressure variables exerted by the various parts of the body on the different areas of the mattress. The trial allows you to determine the ideal support for each customer. Sleep is, therefore, a function of vital importance, like breathing. For this reason, the initiatives of the World Sleep Day will be promoted in all PerDormire stores.

Healthy Sleep, Healthy Aging

World sleep day—is a global event to focus attention on rest, its importance and quality: healthy sleep is essential at any age and, indeed, the quality of life and aging a healthy rest can positively condition it.

Otherwise, disturbed sleep affects daily life, personal health, aging mechanisms, and life quality. The initiative is promoted by the World Sleep Society, the international association committed to the global dissemination of sleep culture and its consequences for our health. The promoting committee, made up of scientists from all over the world, sees two Italians: Liborio Parrino, professor of neurology at the University of Parma—who chairs the committee—and Laura Paladini, psychiatrist of the University hospital of Pisa. An expert in the study of sleep and dreams. The World Sleep Society is attended by a worldwide representation of associations, doctors, and researchers who pool studies and scientific research on sleep, related diseases, and disorders.

Sleep Disorders, Pay Attention

Lack of sleep can seriously undermine our health. According to scientists, a good seven or 8-hour sleep per night is the most important thing we need to do to improve our present and future physical and mental condition. Children need more hours to enjoy the best learning conditions. Why is sleep so important? Recent research indicates that rest is necessary for our brain's health: sleep plays an essential role. In this phase, the synapses—the connections from neuron to neuron—created during the day are readjusted. While you sleep, your brain performs a 'file reset,' eliminating unnecessary processes.

Furthermore, during sleep, neurotoxic substances produced during the day are drained (Dr. Erik St. Louis, Co-Director of the Mayo Center for

Sleep Medicine in Rochester, Minnesota). Assim, the Italian Scientific Association for Research and Education in Sleep Medicine, provides some data that help us to understand the problem: 15% of Italians suffer from chronic insomnia: 25% of road accidents are due to sleepiness; 47% of children sleep less than necessary; 18% of children suffer from sleep-disordered breathing. In addition to clinical sleep problems, some bad habits compromise the quality of our sleep, resulting in a low rate of rest, situations to which, in general, we do not pay too much attention. According to the Sleep Medicine Center of the Niguarda Hospital in Milan, sleep disorders are on the rise, even in the first three years of life, affecting about 30% of families.

Proper Sleep Hygiene: A Suitable Bed and Simple Rules

So, no joking with rest: let's equip ourselves with a quality bed, with ergonomic features suited to our needs, and follow the rules spread by the World Sleep Society: 10 useful tips to ensure a healthy rest for adults.

10 Commandments for Good Sleep Hygiene for Adults

1. Go to bed and wake up at the same time, if possible.

2. If you are in the habit of taking an afternoon nap, don't exceed 45 minutes.

3. Avoid consuming excessive amounts of alcohol in the 4 hours before bedtime, and don't smoke.

4. Avoid taking caffeine in the 6 hours before going to bed; it is present in coffee, tea, many fizzy drinks, chocolate.

5. Avoid eating very spicy or fatty and sweet foods at four o'clock before bedtime. Some light snacks you can eat without overdoing it.

6. Exercise regularly, but not before bed.

7. Use a comfortable, cozy, ergonomically suitable bed.

8. Find a comfortable temperature for your sleep and keep the room well ventilated.

9. Eliminate all noises that may bother you, including light sources.

10. Reserve your bed for sleep and sex. Avoid using it as a workstation or other activities, such as playing video games, eating, watching TV.

A bad habit is enough to disturb sleep and make waking up a real drama. But sleeping better is possible, and nutrition also plays its part!

A troubled night, punctuated by continuous awakenings or periods of insomnia, has the direct consequence of a tiring day to face, with a low level of concentration and a lot of accumulated fatigue. Sleeping well is right for you. It seems like a play on words, but more and more studies confirm that you also need to rest well at night to lead a peaceful and healthy life.

However, we often acquire bad habits over time, which, perhaps even unconsciously, affect our night's rest and, in turn, our daily performance. Better understand immediately what we are doing wrong and run for cover. We have prepared this checklist of 12 good habits to introduce into our life to sleep better and wake up full of energy.

Dinner Yes, But Light

Indeed, you will have noticed, and a too abundant and "heavy" dinner disturbs sleep. Better to have an evening meal based on foods rich in whole carbohydrates (which are assimilated quickly), few proteins, and lightly seasoned vegetables. If possible, the consumption of fats, sugars, and spices should be avoided.

Yes, to Foods That Regulate the Sleep-Wake Rhythm

Foods such as barley, brown rice, tomatoes, corn, oats, oranges, and bananas rich in melatonin, a substance that helps you relax and fall asleep, are recommended for dinner. Foods rich in tryptophan (an essential amino acid that raises serotonin levels in the brain and melatonin), magnesium, and vitamin B are also shown to prevent insomnia, stress, and depression. Therefore, greenlight dried fruit, legumes, ricotta, fish, spinach, and leafy vegetables (for dinner based on salad, choose lettuce, for example).

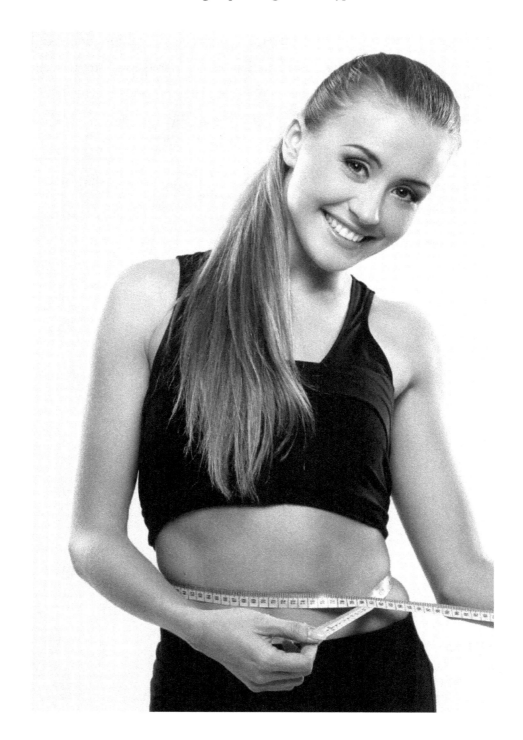

Chapter 8.

Meditation Accessible to All

Being active, doing several things simultaneously, what could be better than a busy life? And when we do nothing or slow down, our little inner voice (mind) calls out to us: "Don't fall behind," "You have to hurry," "There is still that to do." And here we are in "autopilot" mode most of the time, operating without really thinking or understanding what we are doing or why we are doing it.

Trapped in a way by modern life, we forget to introduce a parenthesis into our days and take time to recharge our batteries. Mindful meditation brings this bubble of protection and allows everyone to make this appointment with themselves.

The Benefits of Meditation

Several studies prove that mindfulness meditation regularly allows you to be more present to what you are doing, more attentive to your body, needs, emotions, choices, and listening to others. Its practice allows you to refocus on yourself, your interior space. People who meditate regularly improve their concentration and attention skills. They are calmer, more pleasant, and more tolerant of themselves. They develop a better ability to relax, to manage stressful situations, they have more energy and enthusiasm for life. These people also see a decrease in physical and psychological symptoms related to stress.

How Does Meditation Work?

To meditate means to stop, pose, and observe without judging what is happening inside oneself. It also means listening to what is manifested in you: your thoughts, your emotions, the physical sensations you feel.

Mindful meditation requires focusing on the present moment and allowing yourself to do nothing, not easy when you always have a lot to do!

To help you in the practice of meditation, voluntarily bring your attention to your breathing, a sensation, a part of your body, a physical feeling, a sound, an emotion very gently, without getting carried away by the chattering mind that arises and tries to pull you away from the object of your attention.

A few minutes or even a few seconds of practice is enough to realize how your mind keeps escaping. We think of everything except the object of his attention: in the past tense "I should have done this," "I never succeed," "Why did he tell me that?," or in the future: "I must not forget to go to the store on my way home, "What am I going to tell the chef tomorrow."

Meditation cannot be learned only from a book. It is practiced. And like any new practice, only repetition and training will pay off.

Whatever you choose, "try" is the watchword.

At your own pace, explore the practice of meditation, taking into account your current wishes and your possibilities, without wanting to obtain results at all costs and without wishing to model yourself on a defined practice that imposes a precise timing or posture.

Meditating is a solitary experience, but it is quite possible to join a group to enjoy an atmosphere conducive to meditative work, guided by a trained person and exchanged with other meditators.

Do you prefer to start alone? Start with the exercise suggested below. The important thing is to dare to experience it.

Practice Meditation

Meditation is practiced standing or sitting, eyes open or closed, and even while walking, when you are more trained. Suppose the different forms of meditative practices are infinite and varied

In that case, they have many points in common and often come together in their effects: the presence in the body (and its sensations), the work on breathing, and the concentration on the present moment are some of the keys to meditation.

How a Mindful Breath-Based Meditation Session Works

Start by preparing the equipment for your comfort: a cushion, a blanket, and an outfit in which you are comfortable. Take off your shoes.

Get into a comfortable posture:

Sitting on a chair with your feet flat on the floor, your back slightly off the chair. Seated on the ground on a cushion, legs in lotus for the most flexible.

Laying on the back. Allow yourself to settle in as you see fit.

Set a silent timer (GSM, for example) for the duration you have chosen (a few minutes to start) so that you don't have to think about it anymore.

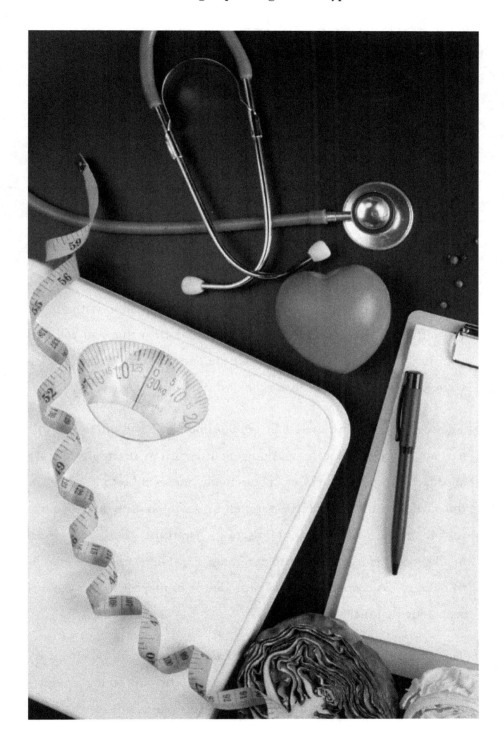

Chapter 9.

Some Keys to Relax

As sales of antidepressants continue to grow, it seems relevant to me to suggest here some other means of regulating your inner tension. Strategies for reducing physical and psychological stress can be grouped into four broad categories.

The first is about solving the problems that create tension. Without any real difficulty to solve, the chances are indeed great that you will find your body relatively relaxed and your mind at ease. Therefore, solving your problems is a way of living the body and mind more relaxed.

The second concerns interior life and attitudes; we will often read that it is not so much the external things that disturb us regarding how we approach them that stress us. The remedy here will be to learn to see things differently: reframing, assertiveness, ability to drop out, cognitive restructuring, behavior modification, spiritual life, emotional intelligence, neurolinguistic programming, etc. There are many schools to help us. To change individual attitudes or to present to our ways of seeing life that make it less trying.

The third grouping of ways to reduce stress focuses on the biochemistry of stress. Here you lower your blood pressure by consuming products with relaxing properties: anxiolytics, antidepressants, muscle relaxants, sleeping pills, alcohol (in small quantities). Finally, the fourth category includes psycho-corporal relaxation strategies. It is what I want to address here briefly.

Relaxation

The avowed goal of relaxation methods is to reduce our state of bodily and psychic tension. In the scientific sense of the term, relaxing is voluntarily devoting time to using a relaxation technique.

This somewhat strict definition does not exclude that other means may give similar results (physical activity, cinema or theater, readings, meeting friends, etc.). It just means that science has confirmed that specific, precise methods bring about beneficial relaxation.

The Eight Ingredients of Relaxation

Each relaxation method is made up of a particular combination of a certain number of the following eight elements: breathing, physical position, voluntary relaxation of the muscles, stretching or massages, concentration, attitude "let-be" (attitude of observation of this happening in his mind), autosuggestion or visualization, and ultimately reduced external stimulation.

Depending on the method, some of these ingredients are more present than others.

For example, hatha-yoga emphasizes breathing, stretching, and voluntary relaxation of the muscles. Autogenic training (Schultz) focuses on voluntary muscle relaxation, concentration, the "let-be" attitude. The autosuggestion and progressive relaxation (Jacobson) offer attention to specific muscle contractions and stretches, all followed by relaxation. Dr. Benson's method is based on voluntary vacation, breathing accompanied by words or sounds, concentration, and the attitude of letting-being. An environment conducive to calm is also a common ingredient in all of the methods mentioned above.

Although each particular method emphasizes certain elements, all have in common to give the same block of results linked to reducing stress, which brings a host of preventive and curative benefits, both in the body and in mind. As the list of these benefits is quite long, I will just say that the practice of relaxation will improve the functioning of everything that reacts badly to stress (concentration, emotional balance, mood, sleep, digestion, cardiovascular, immune, respiratory, digestive, or musculoskeletal systems, etc.). It also has immense preventative benefits because peace works by supporting the mechanisms that keep the body in balance. In fact, in serene and peaceful moments.

Associated Methods

Unlike drugs whose molecules induce artificial changes in the nervous system, relaxation methods only promote a natural reflex's arrival in the body. When, several times a day, our pets abstain from all activity not to sleep but simply relax, they do the same: they rest, as they spontaneously "know" how to do. Relaxation is an organic response like stress or sleep; it occurs naturally when conditions are right. The relaxation methods, therefore, only provide favorable conditions for this organic response.

And since the methods are made up of specific ingredients, everyone could create specific relaxing ways: focusing on music while relaxing their muscles in the bath, aimlessly leafing through books of nature pictures or reproductions. Paintings by the great painters taking care to keep a deep breath, creep, relaxing the back of the neck and shoulders while directing his attention to the images or sounds that reach us and returning to them as soon as his mind begins to "think, "Etc. It would only remain to use his method for about thirty minutes a day, and in all probability, the same results would be obtained as with an official form.

Thirty minutes a day!!! Are you insane? We already don't have time to breathe

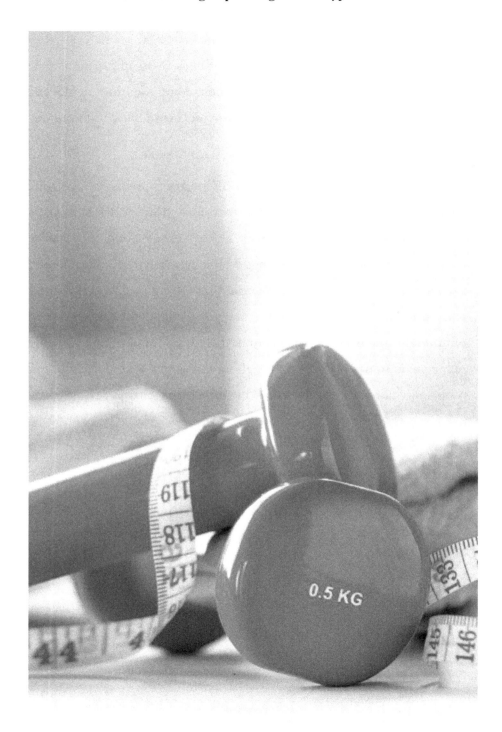

Chapter 10.

Stress Management

We must know and train in a series of techniques that will combat the body's reactions. These reactions can be physiological, emotional, cognitive, and behavioral. If we do not know how to handle and manage them properly, they will produce various clinical manifestations, known to all, which can become chronic and lead to psychosomatic exhaustion. When we come to this type of situation, it is too late. There is scientific evidence of the influence of chronic stress in myocardial infarction, stroke, and weakening of the immune system, among other effects.

In this exhibition, I want to take Seneca as a basis in one of his phrases: "What reason does not achieve, time often performs." With this starting point, I will describe below the twenty techniques that will help us to master stress.

1. Practice Physical Exercise

I fully agree with John F. Kennedy when he stated "physical health is not only one of the most important keys to a healthy body, but the foundation of creative and dynamic intellectual activity." The development and maintenance of good physical condition have very positive effects on the prevention of stress. For this, it is advisable to exercise regularly since, in addition to increasing the physical resistance of the individual to the effects of stress, it enhances psychological resistance. Doing exercise forces us to shift our attention from psychological problems and rest and recover from previously developed mental activity.

Physical exercise mobilizes the body and improves its functioning and physical capacity. Consequently, you will be in better condition to cope with stress, which increases the capacity for physical work and improves cardiovascular, respiratory, and metabolic functions.

In general terms, it can be said that, at present, the professional activity requires fewer and fewer responses of a physical nature and more of an intellectual nature. With exercise, organic resources are used and consumed that can rarely be used to develop a professional activity. If they are not "burned," these resources can be deposited in the vascular system and cause, among other problems, an increase in the level of blood pressure. It is pertinent now to recall a phrase by Edward Stanley: "Those who believe that they do not have time to exercise, sooner or later have to find time to be sick."

2. Proper Diet

The development of good eating habits that determine the individual's nutritional status constitutes an advisable measure for preventing stress.

The energy demands that we currently receive from our environment determine the need to maintain an adequate energy balance to respond to these demands and not develop deficiency problems.

The Mediterranean diet, which is based on olive oil, fruit, cereals, fish, and lean meats, is a crucial aspect of our health. Doug Larson said it: "Life expectancy would increase by leaps and bounds if vegetables smelled as good as bacon."

3. Systematic Desensitization

This technique attempts to control anxiety or fear reactions to situations that are threatening to an individual.

It is based on Jacobson's progressive relaxation, which consists of training the individual in the performance of physical contraction-relaxation exercises.

This action will allow you to know the state of tension of each part of your body and have resources to relax these areas when they are tense.

4. Stress Inoculation

It is a cognitive and behavioral technique. Its methodology is similar to that of systematic desensitization. Starting from learning breathing and relaxation practices to relax tension in stressful situations, the subject creates a list of stressful situations.

5. Physical Relaxation Techniques

The most commonly used are Jacobson's progressive relaxation and Schultz autogenic training. These techniques try to take advantage of the direct connection between the body and the mind, interdependence between psychological and physical tension.

In other words, it is not possible to be physically relaxed while under emotional stress. According to the theories that inspire these techniques, people can learn to reduce their psychological (emotional) tension through physical relaxation, even when the situation that causes the uncertainty persists.

Chapter 11.

Believe in Yourself

How many times have we talked about health on this blog? Today we will talk about a variant that is not discussed very often on this subject of faith. Faith in yourself, believing that you can achieve something in life, have goals and plans, and fulfill dreams. We try too hard to have a healthy body when the state of mind influences a person's well-being exponentially.

As we said at the beginning, healthy life begins when you eat adequate food and love yourself. All extremes are wrong. Don't become obsessed with eating a balanced diet, beating yourself up, and forgetting about your value as a person. Do not look at your cost as a person and your whims, failing your physical health.

"One more day, my alarm goes off at seven in the morning, and as always, my eyes don't even have the strength to open. What am I going to get up for? What will the day offer me differently? Is it better today than tomorrow? What nonsense yesterday was not worth it, today is not going to be different, and hopefully, tomorrow will never come.

I go down to breakfast without wanting anything, thinking about what excuse I'm going to give my mother today for not going to class. I'm not going to waste time trying to get to something that I'm never going to achieve. I will not be able to finish high school or enter the university, nor will they catch me in any job. As soon as I finish breakfast, I go back to bed. I am exhausted. I am awakened by the noise of my best friend's WhatsApp how heavy. Lately, she doesn't stop insisting on seeing us. Will she ever understand that I prefer to be alone at home? It seems that no one understands that I do not want to leave the house that I do not want to see anyone or explain what I feel or think.

No way am I going to go down to eat. Lately, I have been gaining weight because of my sedentary life; But if I'm fatter without eating anything, I'll have to try harder because I'm starting to disgust that's how fast it's expected that no one loves me.

So, without further ado, this has been my day. As I told you, I did not expect anything good or new I go back to bed, in my routine, I hope that tomorrow the alarm clock does not wake me, to suffer again.

"One more day, my alarm goes off at seven in the morning, and as always, I wake up from a jump out of bed. I have math first thing in the morning, my favorite subject, so I don't want to be late.

I go down to breakfast, and on the way, I meet my mother, whom I greeted with a kiss and a good hug yesterday. I did not see her all day. I already wanted to give her my super hug. She has prepared me eggs with bacon to start the day with strength. She is cuter

I get to class, and I meet my best friend. What party yesterday! He starts showing me all the photos we took, and we laugh. With so much joke,

I'm late for math, so I start running through the corridors. I'm a bit lost, so I have to solve a couple of doubts for the exam, that as the average drops a little, I will not enter the race; but the same thing always happens to me the day before the test, it's my nerves I'll end up getting it right.

After class, I'm going to eat with my friends at our usual restaurant they give us incredible discounts, and we eat like kings for something it is our favorite. I go back to bed. What surprises await me tomorrow? Will I pass my math test? You want to start working and university life NOW."

It may sound very abrupt, but these were my thoughts, my days, before entering. I didn't feel like leaving the house, and I didn't want to see or do anything. I couldn't think of tomorrow; I couldn't take this life. I just wanted it to end.

How things change when you believe in yourself. A perfect day begins when you wake up motivated and go to sleep thinking that you will reach your aspirations, how your life changes when you start saying good things to yourself, setting goals and objectives, looking forward to tomorrow, when you begin to love yourself. How much you feel loved, and that you are worth it. When you can criticize yourself in a constructive and non-destructive way, when you can express how you feel, what you think, or what you do without fear of what they will say, you can laugh, cry and scream feel. Be who you want to be. Have fun, enjoy it. Put attitude to life.

Chapter 12.

How to Increase Your Vibration and Stay Away From the Negative Energy of Others?

When dramatic events happen in life, our energies will fluctuate between highs and lows. It can be a challenging adventure to figure out how to get rid of negative energy. Very often, people choose to isolate themselves entirely as self-defense and defend their power. It is not necessary. It's about setting your energy limits. Think of them as locks in your house. Locks, like your energy limits, keep people away until you know that you are safe and secure, and then you can undo the waves and let them in.

Identify Excess Negative Energy

Sometimes we try so hard to be there for others to lose sight of our own needs and ignore the warning signs that negative energy is lowering our overall energetic vibration. Some signs that it is time to raise your vibration and get rid of negative energy are:

- Mood swings

- Apathy

- Fatigue

- Loss of concentration

- Anxiety

- Restlessness

- Physical pain such as headaches, stomach aches, even chest pains

How to Get Rid of Negative Energy?

Eliminate clutter, physical and spiritual. Clean spaces and open spaces in your living area can give you peace of mind and serenity.

Purge emotional clutter like trapped emotions.

Literally, "bury" yourself. This concept is also known as "grounding." Do you know what a great feeling you have after a day at the beach? That is more than a relaxing day.

Standing or walking barefoot on grass, sand, or even a concrete surface immediately above the ground can release increasingly damaging negative energy from your body.

Mindfulness and Eating Disorders

Mindfulness is a relaxation technique that teaches us to become fully aware of our emotions.

Several scientific studies have shown the benefits of mindfulness for the treatment of eating disorders. In recent years, the practice of mindfulness (also called mindfulness) has been gained followers.

It is a relaxation technique that teaches us to become fully aware of our emotions and is based mainly on:

Self-observation of body exploration, which allows us to become aware of our sensations.

Meditation, with particular emphasis on the present and on the connection between body and mind. Mindfulness in everyday life consists of paying attention to all thoughts and feelings, without judging whether they are good or bad: just observing them.

Stretches and YOGA

In the 1970s, Dr. Jon Kabat-Zinn of Massachusetts University in the U.S. developed the "Mindfulness-Based Stress Reduction" (MBSR) program. It is a training in which mindfulness is applied to treat certain physical and mental conditions as a complementary route to traditional treatments.

Since then, interest in the clinical application of mindfulness has been growing, so the scientific community has seen the need to study the impact of this technique on different diseases or conditions and on eating disorders such as anorexia bulimia.

Mindfulness and Eating Disorders

A study published in the journal Health Promotion assessed the impact of an online feeding and mindfulness program.

This initiative, called "Eat for Life," aimed to instruct people with eating disorders in the practice of mindfulness.

The study authors randomly distributed participants into two groups: one participated in the Eat for Life program, and the other did not.

After ten weeks, both groups had significant differences in symptoms. The group that had performed the intuitive mindfulness-based feeding program was 3.65 times more likely to become asymptomatic, i.e., not to have symptoms of eating disorders concerning the other group.

More and more studies are being done that, like this one, evaluate the application of mindfulness in eating disorders. While more data is still needed, mindfulness-based interventions are beginning to be seen in combination with other strategies such as food-oriented behavioral therapies are an effective alternative to improving symptoms.

What Are the Benefits of Mindfulness In Eating Disorders?

According to studies, the practice of mindfulness results in an improvement in symptoms of eating disorders in the following aspects:

- Emotional management skills

- The relationship with food

- Own perception of bodily sensations, learning to distinguish between real and emotional hunger

- Behavioral improvements, with the normalization of eating habits

- Resetting the weight

All these studies motivate the development of programs that use such practices for the treatment of eating disorders. However, scientists stress that more studies are needed to confirm the effectiveness and provide guidelines for designing effective interventions.

Chapter 13.

Exercise—The Mind and Body

A different technique to feel better thanks to yoga. Benefits of eating disorders.

For the treatment of anorexia and bulimia, a multidisciplinary intervention has always been proposed to incorporate new techniques that favor the process.

One of these techniques is Yoga. Several studies have shown how yoga is very favorable. It promotes patients to feel better about their bodies, better capture their physical sensations, healthier attitudes towards food, and feeling more satisfied with themselves, and decrease the figure's anxiety.

Studies have also shown how yoga has more positive therapeutic effects on eating disorders than other sports practices (such as running).

Kundalini Yoga

There are several different types of Yoga, one of which is Kundalini. It is characterized by combining physical exercises, mental concentration, breathing techniques, relaxation, and meditation, promoting physical and psychological health. It also encourages the person to connect with aspects of himself other than appearance and personality.

Meditation, as part of this technique, is one of the fundamental pillars, as it promotes greater control over the mind by observing the contents of consciousness, so it implies a strategy of dominance and self-control. Numerous studies conducted with meditation have found that it increases psychological well-being, decreases anxiety, improves emotional regulation, and raises awareness and body acceptance, thus improving life quality.

Yoga is a practice that decreases anxiety and negative thoughts and increases the feeling of self-control. This is because, under anxious states, reviews are becoming faster and faster. However, while yoga is being exercised, the concentration lies in breathing and the body, returning attention to the present moment. This causes negative thought patterns to decrease, becoming slower and more conscious for the person.

Shift towards a Positive Vision

After a study of 9 eating disorder patients practicing Kundalini Yoga, they found that a more positive view of life arose in several aspects:

More extraordinary ability to be in the present, of personal time and of being with themselves: "I've been enjoying being with me, I didn't like it before... But I've started to have a good time and feel more cheerful..."

Feeling of gratitude and appreciation for one's life: "...Acceptance of diversity that we were all different and everything I had done was perfect," "...Acceptance of who I am, and thank the universe for it...The universe loves us, it loves me! That's what I've been feeling."

They increased self-assessment in various factors, such as decreased external judgment, a sense of greater capacity and personal safety, greater sociability, greater capacity for self-preservation and internal contact, more effective self-assessment and awareness, acceptance of one's own body, and positive contact with one's femininity.

Changes in the emotional experience also emerged, as feelings and emotions of personal well-being increased (expressing more happiness, calm, balance, fullness, love, satisfaction, pleasure, vitality, and freedom). Besides, it changed the way they spoke and endured unpleasant emotions,

On the other hand, participants developed different personal capacities, such as exercising greater self-control over the symptomatology of the disease (expressed in increasing alternative behaviors, increased awareness of food intake, or the emergence of positive sensations and attitudes towards food), as well as a development of the ability to establish limits of their own towards others or a change of attitude towards conflict (distance capacity and better confrontation). Finally, a positive difference in the content of thoughts, manifested in a greater awareness of them, and with the appearance of views contrary to disorder.

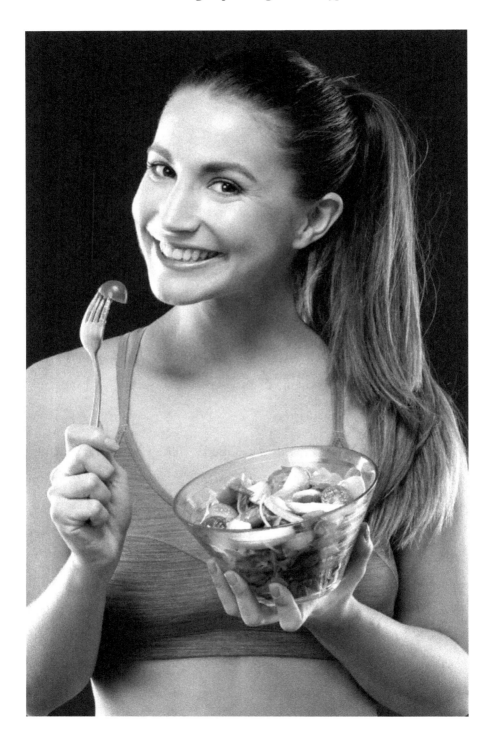

Chapter 14.

Yoga to Treat Eating Disorders

A ll that interferes with regular nutrient intake and produces different consequences that are generally not beneficial to health are eating disorders.

Fortunately, it is possible to resort to yoga to treat eating disorders, as we tell you in this article of "Other Medicine."

How Yoga Will Help You with Eating Disorders

When you have these types of food problems, whether it's bulimia, anorexia, or both at the same time, a low diet usually influences the mind-body relationship.

Thanks to yoga, you will learn to listen to your body and build a consciousness to understand what is happening to you and find a solution.

Yoga will also help you focus your attention on your health and not so much on your appearance. It is very likely that, over time, by practicing this discipline, you will learn to listen to your interior and not so much to look at your exterior appearance.

It Will Gives You Muscle Memory

Muscle, believe it or not, has a strong memory. With this discipline's regular practice, you will teach your body to form a kind of muscle memory that will have a significant and positive impact on your figure.

This will mean that it will be much easier for you to achieve yoga asanas and, in this way, not resort to counterproductive food practices.

A Holistic Approach Is Achieved

Using yoga and meditation, you will treat eating problems through a holistic approach because it connects the mind and body, giving you the serenity necessary to face eating disorders with a calm mind.

This is extremely useful as most eating problems originate in the mind and body distortion that those suffering from this type of disease see in front of the mirror.

The main factors in eating disorders, as I mentioned above, occur in the mind, but are a sum of several factors, including the psychological part, behavior, social, or merely biological causes.

According to studies of patients with eating disorders, yoga has a tremendously positive effect on depression, low self-esteem, anxiety, and anger.

It will also help you create healthy habits, order your meals, and understand much more clearly that it is possible to get out of this disease and return to everyday life. Tell us, do you practice yoga? Is that useful to you?

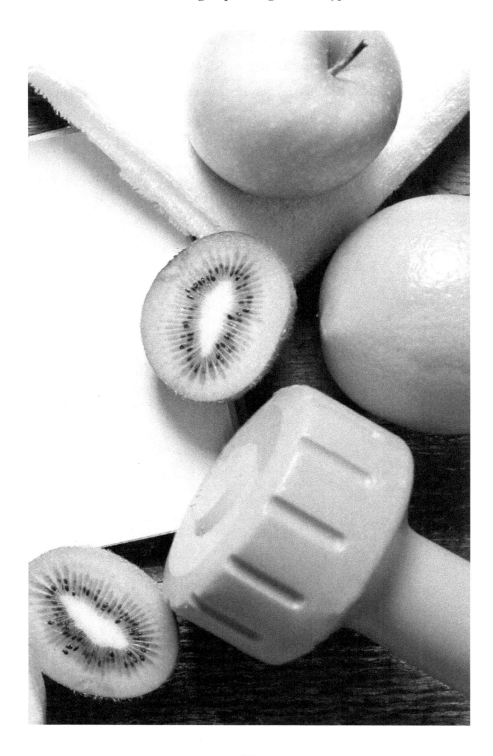

Chapter 15.

Mindfulness for Food Disorders

When food becomes the center of life, you are faced with an eating disorder that hides emotional problems.

Mindfulness is a powerful tool, recognized as an effective way to reduce stress, increase self-awareness, reduce physical and psychological symptoms associated with stress, and improve overall well-being.

Although the practice of mindfulness has recently been integrated into medicine and psychology in the world's leading universities and medical centers, it is an ancient practice that originates more than 2,500 years ago with Buddhism.

Mindfulness means to consciously pay attention to the present moment's experience with interest, curiosity, and acceptance. Jon Kabat-Zinn is known as his world leader for introducing this practice into the Western medical model more than 30 years ago.

There is a disorder in eating behavior when a person's attitudes toward food and weight are such that feelings toward work, study, relationships, and daily activities are determined by what has or has not been eaten or by a number on the scale (Siegel, Bris man, and Weinshal).

The person who suffers from an eating behavior disorder is characterized by being an extremist in terms of food consumption, manifested by severe weight loss, rapid weight gains, or very significant fluctuations in it.

He is disgusted with his body image, often accompanied by a distorted perception of the body's signals (hunger, anger, fatigue, etc.).

It is common for this person to perform unhealthy practices to maintain weight: fasting, starvation, compulsive eating, indiscriminate use of laxatives, or other medications for weight loss and excess exercise, including. The three most common disorders, sorted by frequency, are binge eating, bulimia nervosa, and anorexia nervosa.

Incidence

Anyone can have an eating disorder, which usually occurs between 12 and 25, although there are exceptions in both directions. 90% occur in women and 10% in men.

They tend to appear when the person suffering from it is going through a difficult period of transition, shock, or loss.

Food behavior disorders are governed by a deficit in the identification and management of emotions and in the regulation that the person makes in his food intake. Food intake self-regulation disorder is linked to difficulty recognizing the physiological signs of hunger and satiety and discerning these signals from the body's signals of each emotion.

Mindfulness approaches can intervene by improving self-regulation, and evidence begins to emerge that demonstrates its potential usefulness.

Duke University's Jean Kristeller is co-founder of The Center for Mindful Eating (www.tcme.org), a non-profit entity engaged in the training and disseminating mindfulness practice to eating disorders.

Among the principles Kristeller recommends are:

1- Observe without judging the very reactivity of behavior (a load of thoughts, emotions, and physical sensations that govern behavior).

2- Separate emotions from this load and learn that emotions are common facts that often do not require a response (the disorder of emotions regulation reflects deficits when identifying, managing, and adaptively using emotions).

3- Separate thoughts from this burden of reactivity and learn that thoughts are just thoughts, passenger facts that often do not require an answer.

4- Separate and tolerate behavioral impulses from that load of reactivity.

5- Reconnect and relink "in a simple way" with the physiological signs of hunger and satiety (gastric satiety).

6- Pay attention to the specific satiety of taste.

7- Distinguish corporeal sensations from emotions, and discern indications of appetite regulation.

8- Identify actual needs ("Am I famished?").

9- Wise and informed decision-making to fill the real need. (Stop—Breathe—Connect).

Confinement and Food Behavior Disorders

During confinement, boredom and anxiety can complicate Food Behavior Disorders' treatment and lead to a change in people's diet. The feeling of being out of the house, as during confinement, can increase obsessive thinking about food. Too much free time can lead to a cycle of food binge bingeing due to anxiety and boredom, which can worsen ADHD.

Food Behavior Disorders: What Are They?

Food Behavior Disorders (ACS) are "mental disorders characterized by pathological behavior in the face of food intake and an obsession with weight management," according to the Association against Anorexia and Bulimia.

Some of these disorders include:

- Anorexia nervosa: fear of gaining weight, as a consequence, restrict your caloric intake.

- Bulimia: the presence of self-induced binge and subsequent vomiting or other purging maneuvers.

- Binge disorder: episodes of compulsive intake repeatedly.

- Bigorexia: an obsession with physical exercise.

- Orthorexia: an obsession with healthy food.

According to data from the Fita Foundation, approximately 400,000 people in Spain have anorexia nervosa, bulimia, or binge eating disorder. The vast majority of these people are young women, especially pre-teens and adolescents. These disorders are severe if not treated but can be solved if they perform treatment and follow-up with a team of specialized doctors and psychologists.

Chapter 16.

Food and Mental Health

A bibliographic review captures the primary nutrients that affect proper brain development and the impact of the nutritional deficit on disorders such as depression. The brain is the organ that requires the most energy: it absorbs between 20% and 27% of the body's metabolic rate. That's why it needs nutrients for proper functioning and development. In this way, the nutrient deficit can have consequences on mental health. Studies associate the role of nutrients with behavioral and cognitive manifestations in depression or mood disorders.

A bibliographic review discusses the importance of various nutrients in brain function and the development of mental illnesses such as depression. The methodology used has been a systematic review of the literature on nutrient deficiency's psychological and neurological effects. These nutrients are essential fatty acids, folate and vitamin B12, antioxidants, selenium, zinc, and iron.

First, the analysis notes that a diet rich in essential fatty acids decreases the risk of depression, as high concentrations of DHA (an omega-3 fatty acid) increase the sensitivity of Serotonin receptors, the happiness hormone. On the other hand, patients with diseases or mood disorders have been found to have a low concentration of folate and vitamin B12, essential nutrients for the central nervous system.

Selenium also acts as a mood modulator: a deficiency of this nutrient has been observed to reduce immune function, and patients report more symptoms of depression and hostility.

Other studies have shown that individuals with depression have a lower concentration of zinc in their blood. Finally, it has been observed that lack of iron can decrease the enzymes needed for the synthesis and function of dopamine, serotonin, and norepinephrine, which may involve fatigue, irritability, apathy, and lack of concentration.

In conclusion, this determines that nutritional deficiency is common in people with depression and that an improved diet can positively impact anti-depressive therapeutic efficacy. However, it is also stated that the articles analyzed have only studied the impact of food on mental illness in cases with high nutritional deficiency.

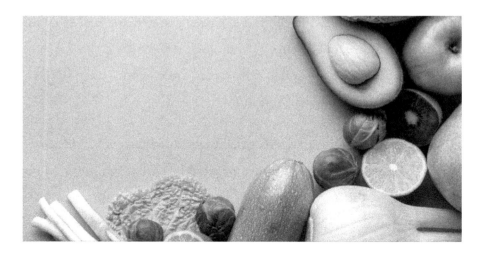

Conclusion

Hypnosis is a state of absorption and internal concentration, such as being in a trance. Hypnosis is usually performed with the help of a hypnotherapist through oral repetition and mental imaging.

When you're under hypnosis, your attention is highly focused, and you respond better to suggestions, including behavioral changes that can help you lose weight.

Some studies have evaluated the use of hypnosis for weight loss. Most studies showed only mild weight loss, with an average loss of approximately 6 pounds (2.7 kilograms) over 18 months. However, the quality of some of these studies has been questioned, making it challenging to determine hypnosis's actual effectiveness for weight loss.

However, a recent study, which showed only modest weight loss results, found that patients receiving hypnosis had lower rates of inflammation, better satiety, and better quality of life. These could be mechanisms by which hypnosis could influence weight. Additional studies are needed to understand the potential role of hypnosis in weight management fully.

CPSIA information can be obtained
at www.ICGtesting.com
Printed in the USA
LVHW081608120621
690059LV00002B/235